SAFFRON HOOTON

Strong Woman Era

HOW TO EMBRACE
YOUR STRENGTH AND
ELEVATE YOUR LIFE

vie

STRONG WOMAN ERA

An Hachette UK Company
www.hachette.co.uk

Vie Books, an imprint of Summersdale Publishers
Part of Octopus Publishing Group Limited
Carmelite House
50 Victoria Embankment
LONDON
EC4Y 0DZ
UK

www.summersdale.com

This FSC® label means that materials used for the product have been responsibly sourced

MIX
Paper | Supporting responsible forestry
FSC® C018236

The authorized representative in the EEA is Hachette Ireland, 8 Castlecourt Centre, Dublin 15, D15 XTP3, Ireland (email: info@hbgi.ie)

Printed and bound in Poland

ISBN: 978-1-83799-492-2

Substantial discounts on bulk quantities of Summersdale books are available to corporations, professional associations and other organizations. For details contact general enquiries: telephone: +44 (0) 1243 771107 or email: enquiries@summersdale.com.

Contents

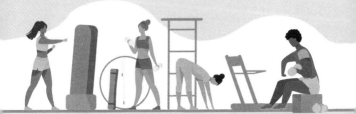

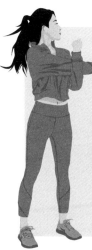

Disclaimer

Neither the author nor the publisher can be held responsible for any injury, loss or claim – be it health, financial or otherwise – arising out of the use, or misuse, of the suggestions made herein. Always consult your doctor before trying any new form of exercise if you have a medical or health condition, or are worried about any of the side effects. This book is not intended as a substitute for the medical advice of a doctor or physician.

STRENGTH TRAINING

/strɛŋθ ˈtreɪnɪŋ/

*Resistance training. Weight training.
Lifting weights.*

The performance of exercises against
a resisting force.

"[Name]'s really into strength training.
She's in her strong woman era."

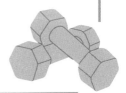

INTRODUCTION

Welcome to your *Strong Woman Era*: a new phase of growth, opportunity and success. This bold book will accompany you on your wellness and weightlifting journey as you harness your mental and physical strength and build your best life.

To understand the relationship between strength training and well-being, let's first consider what "wellness" means. Dr Margaret Swarbrick's model separates wellness into eight dimensions (in no particular order): physical, intellectual, emotional, financial, environmental, occupational, spiritual and social. Total wellness is the integration of these areas: challenging our bodies, engaging our minds and nurturing our spirits.

We know movement is part of what makes us human – with our primate ancestors evolving into endurance runners to increase their chances of survival – and is one of our basic physical and psychological needs. In modern times, our instinct to move can be satisfied in many ways, like by lifting weights. Strength training, meaning the performance of exercises against a resisting force, also supports many of the eight dimensions. In this way we can acknowledge strength training as a key wellness practice, improving our physical, intellectual, emotional and spiritual health.

We can also identify strong as a state of being – it's who we are. Resistance training enables us to tap into our strength, collaborate with our minds and bodies, and realize our capabilities. The practice of strength training is about more than our health; it's about women rising and thriving. Through the act of lifting weights, we confirm that being strong is in our nature: primal, powerful and positively female.

As you move through this book, from starting out with strength training to seeing progress and committing to the lifestyle, you'll discover you are the champion of your health and happiness – this is *your* journey. Now to embrace your authentic self: strong woman.

Discovering Your Strength

What does "strong" mean to you? Is it an appearance, an attitude, an act? The truth is, strong goes beyond how someone looks, the way they behave or a practice they perform; strong is a state of mind.

As women, there are endless ways we can channel our strength: taking action, being passionate, speaking our minds, pursuing our dreams, being unapologetic, taking up space and prioritizing our health and happiness. This journey is about reclaiming our strength and empowering ourselves through wellness practices so that we can live our best lives.

This chapter will introduce the practice of resistance training, discuss the mental and physical benefits of lifting weights, tackle gymtimidation and finding motivation, shed light on the history of female sport, dispel female fitness myths and reframe your mindset to help you discover your strength. It's all about embracing your power, tailoring your approach and celebrating your unique journey.

There isn't one way to look, act or be strong; you simply *are*. It's the dawn of a new era – time for you to discover your strength.

THE KEY TO DISCOVERING YOUR STRENGTH

Before we get started, let's make one thing absolutely clear: you *are* strong. You already have the strength you need to navigate your life and you are more than capable of achieving everything you want to.

But it's also true that sometimes you might not feel so strong. You may sometimes face difficult situations or troubling thoughts that prevent you from speaking up, joining in and doing the things you'd like to do. The good news is, you can incorporate practices into your day that remind you of your strength and enable you to live your best life. One of these practices is strength training.

Strength training can ground you in your body and encourage you to be in the present moment. It focuses your mind, expels the thoughts that don't serve you, and makes you appreciate just how much you can do.

It can be incredibly empowering to move your body in new and challenging ways and accomplish feats you didn't think were possible. Lifting weights validates your tenacity, your drive and your ability to overcome obstacles, helping you recognize how powerful you are.

The practice of strength training can also inspire you to pursue your own growth and development and strive for success in other areas of your life. It enhances the relationship you have with yourself and improves your understanding of your own needs, helping you trust, respect and honour your body.

The feelings of pride, satisfaction and self-appreciation that training brings continue well beyond your workouts and help you foster a more positive mindset. When you feel low, you can remind yourself of your value, how competent you are and how committed you are to your health and happiness.

Strength training is not about transforming yourself into someone that you're not, because you are worthy of love, kindness and admiration exactly as you are. It's about helping you recognize your strength, harness your power and prove to yourself that you deserve the life you want.

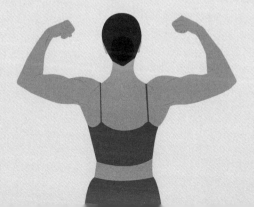

THE FEMALE INCENTIVE

Movement is a part of being human and is integral to our well-being, but why would we, as women, choose strength training over other forms of exercise? Well, because we can! And because, although the practice can seem male-dominated, there are many mental and physical benefits specifically for women. Understanding these can incentivize us to commit to our wellness journeys.

Beyond the greater impact of feeling strong, resistance training enables us to physically thrive; it increases the size, tone and strength of our muscles, improves our cardiovascular (heart and lung) health, reduces our blood pressure, stabilizes and protects our joints, raises our metabolic rate, enhances our body composition, promotes greater mobility and flexibility, and helps us sleep better.

For women in particular, weight-bearing exercise increases our bone density – something that peaks around the age of 30 and decreases sharply during the menopause. Being female automatically puts us at greater risk of osteoporosis, but we can build strong bones and slow bone loss through strength training.

Research also suggests that physical activity can positively impact the strength and function of the pelvic floor muscles. These muscles support the bladder, uterus and bowel, as well as help us have better sex, so it's essential we train them regularly.

Weight training is not only brilliant for our physical strength; it's also a powerful tool to help improve our mental health. Exercise can elevate our mood, increase our body confidence, raise our self-esteem, combat feelings of stress and improve cognitive function. Studies in England show that women are twice as likely as men to be diagnosed with anxiety, with 62 per cent of females also reporting that they feel negatively about their body image. Because of this, it's especially important that we as women actively protect and nurture our headspace.

Through strength training, we can boost our mental state, break the bias and build ourselves up at the same time.

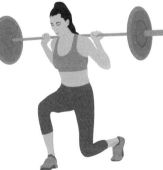

I am a woman

phenomenally.

Phenomenal

woman,

that's me.

MAYA ANGELOU

Affirmations

Affirmations are positive statements we can practise daily to promote self-confidence, self-belief and strength. Like resistance training, they help us connect with our power and drive change in our lives. Our thoughts directly affect the way we feel about ourselves – by regularly repeating affirmations, in our heads or aloud, we accept them into our subconscious minds.

Practise these as part of your morning routine:

I love myself, I believe in myself, I belong.

I am protected, I am guided.

*I release thoughts and feelings
that do not serve me.*

I welcome opportunities for growth.

I have everything I need within me to succeed.

*I am grateful for who I am
and who I'm becoming.*

The Power of Strength Training

There are numerous practices that benefit our well-being. To understand the role of exercise in our wellness journeys, we need to consider the relationship between resistance training and other aspects of our health.

Strength training is only one form of exercise – however you choose to move your body counts towards your well-being.

While exercise can help reduce feelings of stress, talking therapy is often a useful tool for managing anxiety.

Working out will help you build the foundations of a healthy routine, but finding time for self-care and socializing makes for a healthy lifestyle.

Weight training will help you recognize how strong and capable you are, but affirmations and positive self-talk reinforce the message.

Lifting weights will improve your strength, but mobility and flexibility training are essential practices for overall better movement.

Strength training will help you grow muscle and develop shape, but nutrition is key to this process.

Resistance training will yield the greatest results if you prioritize rest and recovery.

Strength training won't make your body more worthy of love; it already deserves it.

Movement can inspire feelings of gratitude for your body and everything it can do, and journalling can help you feel grateful for your life and everything you've achieved.

Training won't "fix" everything, but it will give you more control over your health and happiness which will in turn make a positive impact on your life.

BINNING THE COOKIE CUTTER

We are all unique, and that's a pretty special thing. This individuality makes us powerful, our minds and bodies sacred and our lives incredibly precious.

How our bodies respond to exercise is also completely unique, meaning our approach should be too. We would never look the same as each other even if we followed the same workout routines, ate the same food and led similar lifestyles. The truth is, strength training can't give you someone else's physique, but it can enhance your own.

Our uniqueness is in our DNA, with research showing that our genes can determine up to 80 per cent of our bodies. Understanding this can help us appreciate ourselves and our individual journeys that much more.

Genetic potential refers to someone's ability to put on muscle mass and their natural capacity for physical strength. We can maximize our genetic potential through targeted training and nutrition, but we can't exceed it.

Our genes also determine our body type, height, basal metabolic rate (the calories we burn just by existing) and the nutrients we absorb from food, all of which can impact our approach. Even our proportions will change the way we train; for example, depending on the length of our femurs (thigh bones), our squat form will naturally be more or less upright (see page 130 for how to squat). To discover our true strength, we have to identify and accommodate these differences.

It's not just our bodies, either. In addition to our own lived experiences, our genes also influence the development and function of our brains, our psychological responses, our moods and our behaviours. Taking the time to learn and understand our triggers, our thinking patterns and our reactions can better equip us to establish and maintain positive mental health.

The practices we engage with to support our mental and physical well-being should reflect our individuality. The cookie-cutter approach to health assumes we're all the same when, really, we're one of a kind.

BY CHOOSING TO MOVE EVERY DAY, YOU REAFFIRM YOUR SELF-WORTH

INVESTING IN YOU

One thing you can do every day to champion your strength is choose yourself: choose your happiness, your health and the things that fulfil you and bring you joy.

"Investing in you" means acknowledging how worthy of love, effort and success you are. It means that you believe in yourself so strongly and value yourself so deeply that you put your energy into your mental and physical well-being.

To do this, you could practise mental wellness techniques, such as mindfulness (see page 108), move your body daily, fuel yourself with nutritious food and complete acts of self-love – whatever you feel will benefit you.

You are entitled to set boundaries and be discerning with who and what deserves your time and attention. Do not compromise your mental peace, emotional well-being or any other aspect of your health for the sake of others. To be your strongest, you have to choose yourself.

Listening to Your Body

Your body contains millions of receptors that detect different states, such as hunger, fatigue and stress. These receptors send signals to the brain, alerting it to your needs. It's your responsibility to then listen to your body and identify what you can do to honour your health and support your strength.

Listen: Pay attention to how you're feeling. Tune in to your body, perhaps by closing your eyes and taking several deep breaths.

Identify: Acknowledge what would help you navigate this feeling.

Honour: Action the measure that addresses your needs and supports your total wellness.

Hearing what your body is telling you and responding accordingly helps develop the relationship you have with yourself. You will become more confident in your ability to discern what you actually need and learn to trust yourself when it comes to prioritizing your well-being.

By listening to your body you can start working with it, granting it space in your life and confirming that it is valid and worthy of respect.

Breathwork

We can use our breath to navigate feelings of anxiety, and also to enhance our performance while strength training. Try these techniques:

To feel still

- **Box breathing:** Breathe in for 4 seconds, hold for 4, breathe out for 4, hold for 4.
- **Belly breathing:** Breathe in through your nose, allow your stomach to expand, breathe out through pursed lips, feel your stomach contract.

To feel strong

- **The "effort":** Breathe out through your mouth with the "effort" of the movement, e.g. breathe out as you stand up from a squat.
- **The Valsalva manoeuvre:** Breathe into your stomach and hold this for the duration of the movement, e.g. breathe out at the top of a squat.

TAKING UP SPACE

Women can sometimes feel anxious about metaphorically and physically taking up space, and we often feel compelled to shrink ourselves. Training helps remind us of our strength and the power we possess.

A gym is just one example of where women are taking up space. Although often considered a male-dominated environment, women now make up 54 per cent of gym memberships in the UK, with female strength training growing increasingly accessible and popular.

Gyms are not just for men, or for serious athletes, or for people who are *really* into training. It doesn't matter how long we've been exercising for, how we choose to work out or how much we know about lifting weights; we're entitled to use that space just as much as anyone else. There's no such thing as the men's area, male weights or male equipment – strength is for all.

We can be "big", we can be authentically ourselves and we can be emboldened by the fact that we belong.

Be bold,

be proud

and allow

yourself

to thrive

CONQUERING GYMTIMIDATION

The gym can seem like a scary place – we might feel like we're being judged or that we don't belong. This phenomenon is called gymtimidation, or gym anxiety, and it's experienced by 60 per cent of women, posing a barrier to many of us who would like to pursue our wellness goals.

The truth is, women *do* belong in gyms. It's a space we too can use to move our bodies, improve our mental health and foster feelings of self-love. Everyone's there to work on themselves, so no one's actually watching us! However, if the feeling persists, these tips can help you manage gymtimidation:

1 **Find your space:** Set yourself up somewhere more private. You could take the equipment you need to a quiet corner or studio and complete an effective workout using only dumbbells, for example. Headphones can also help you immerse yourself in your space.

2 **Train at quiet times:** Exercising outside of peak hours and avoiding the pre- and post-work rushes often lends itself to quieter sessions with a greater selection of equipment. Friday evenings, Saturday afternoons and Sundays are usually the least busy times to train.

3   **Bring a friend:** Training with a friend can instantly make you feel more confident. You may have different abilities and goals, and follow your own routines, but it's still nice to see a friendly face in the gym.

4   **Learn staple exercises:** Knowing some key exercises (see pages 130–151) can help you feel more skilled and confident in your training.

5   **Follow a routine:** Having a pre-planned workout routine (plus alternative exercises to fall back on if certain equipment is in use) means you'll know exactly what you're doing, where you're training and what equipment you'll need. This will reduce the overwhelming amount of exercise options you have and help focus your sessions.

6   **Remove the pressure:** If you feel obliged to look and train a certain way, it can increase feelings of gym anxiety. Instead, remember that how you choose to move your body and how you look are valid.

The History of Female Strength

Strong women have always existed; studies into prehistoric female bones show these women regularly practised load-bearing activities, with their arms resembling elite rowers' and their legs similar to those of ultramarathon runners.

Spartan women were known for their strength: Cynisca, a Spartan princess and athlete, became the first woman ever to win an event at the male-only Olympic Games in 396 BCE. Women in ancient Greece also celebrated female agility by competing in the Heraean Games, an event that was considered a rite of passage into womanhood.

Three pioneers of female strength emerged in the Victorian era: Katie Sandwina (whose name was rumoured to have come from defeating the bodybuilder Eugen Sandow), Vulcana (who famously freed a stuck wagon by picking it up) and Minerva. After lifting a platform balancing 23 men, Minerva was awarded the title of the World's Strongest Woman. These women, along with other female lifters at the time, promoted the message that strength, muscularity and femininity could coexist, disputing body ideals we still face today.

Another pioneer of strength sports for women, Ivy Russell, popularized female weight training in Britain before the Second World War. She could deadlift (see page 136) three times her bodyweight, she petitioned for the British Amateur Weightlifting Association to sanction contests for women, and she redefined conventional notions of womanhood.

Abbye (Pudgy) Stockton paved a similar path in America, becoming the first female bodybuilding champion and writing a regular column called "Barbelles". She continued to inspire women in the 1960s and 1970s to challenge claims that female bodies were inferior.

One of these inspired women, powerlifter Jan Todd, lifted a total of 544 kg (1,200 lb) in a competition in 1979, acknowledging "Strength should be an attribute of all humanity. It's not a gift that belongs solely to the male species."

Exercise has never been exclusively for men, and these women in history set about challenging the patriarchal narrative. Like these examples, we too can discover our strength through resistance training. Women have always been and continue to be strong.

There is no limit
to what we,
as women,
can accomplish.

MICHELLE OBAMA

FINDING MOTIVATION

It can be challenging to find the motivation to start strength training, and, once you've started, it's sometimes difficult to stay motivated. Feeling inspired is part of the process of discovering your strength.

These tips can help you find your motivation:

- **Visualize the future:** Consider your goals and imagine how you'll feel when you achieve them. Break them down into smaller steps so they feel more manageable.
- **Channel positive vibes:** Create a motivational atmosphere. Play inspirational music to "hype" yourself up.
- **Plan ahead:** Schedule your sessions. Set out anything you'll need ahead of time and plan a "reward" for after.
- **Reflect:** Acknowledge your journey so far. Remember that setbacks don't mean you're at square one.
- **Just show up:** Turning up is half the battle. Just starting can sometimes be all you need.
- **Make it part of your routine:** Motivation can fail you, but that's when habit kicks in. On average, it takes two months for a behaviour to become automatic and for strength training to become your constant.

DOING WHAT YOU LOVE

What makes you feel strong? Running, swimming, cycling, dancing, strength training... what forms of movement do you enjoy?

A helpful aim for every part of your wellness journey is to come from a place of love: *"I love what I'm doing. I'm doing it because I love myself."* Your priority should always be your health – so you should choose to move your body in ways that make you feel good. Investing in movement that brings you joy is more fulfilling and, when you enjoy what you're doing, you're more likely to commit to it.

It's important to note that all forms of movement are valid. There's no hierarchy when it comes to how you choose to exercise nor is there one "right" way to train. Anything that gets you moving, challenges your body and elevates your heart rate counts.

While this book focuses on resistance training in the "traditional" sense, activities such as Pilates, Barre and pole fitness also require great amounts of strength and offer many of the same benefits as lifting weights (see pages 12–13). Other forms of strength training include powerlifting (weight training focused on squat, bench press and deadlift movements), Olympic lifting (weight training focused on clean and jerk and snatch movements),

Strongwoman (a collection of varied, heavy lifts), Hyrox (a combination of running and functional strength exercises) and bodybuilding (weight training focused on shaping the physique).

Some of the most popular sports across the globe include football, tennis and cricket. There are also more obscure forms of movement, such as chess boxing, mermaiding and toe wrestling. More recently, activities like wild swimming, barefoot running and martial arts have become popular, new sports like pickleball and padel have been created, and "breaking" (an urban dance style) made its Olympic debut in 2024.

Discovering your strength is about finding ways to move that empower you. Do what you love, and love feeling strong.

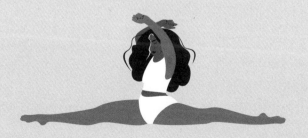

The Evolution of Female Fitness

Strength training is only the latest fitness movement women are redefining. In fact, women have been practising being strong for millennia:

- **5000–2000 BCE:** Tsu Chu and other ball games.

- **1700–1899:** Women compete in sports including boxing, cricket, horse racing, golf, baseball and football.

- **1900–20:** Stretching, exercising using stationary bikes and rowing machines. Also during this time, women's events are introduced into the Olympics.

- **1930–40:** Bodyweight workouts and aerobic dancing.

- **1950–60:** Hula-hooping, twisting and callisthenics.

- **1970–80:** Jogging, Jazzercise, aerobic dancing, Pilates and bodybuilding.

- **1990–2000:** Step aerobics, Tae Bo, spinning, Barre and Zumba.

- **2010s:** Modern yoga, CrossFit and fitness classes.

- **2020s:** Group training, circuit and interval training, Hyrox and strength training.

Daily Walk

A brisk, 30-minute walk offers many mental and physical health benefits, including boosting our mood, improving balance and strengthening our bodies. It's a go-to activity for recovery on days off from resistance training, and a daily walk can be a simple place to start our exercise regimes.

We can approach walking in different ways:

- **Power:** Walking quickly with bent arms improves our cardiovascular fitness and can lower blood pressure.

- **Backwards:** Reverse walking improves our coordination and can ease back and knee pain.

- **Trail:** Trail walking trains our stability and the exposure to nature can alleviate stress.

- **Hill:** Hill walking improves our endurance and stamina, and activates our hamstring, glute and calf muscles.

- **Crab:** Walking sideways improves our ankle and hip stability and strengthens our core and glute muscles.

- **Monster:** Taking small steps forwards while in a squat position activates our hip and glute muscles.

Treating Yourself with Kindness

You deserve kindness – it's as simple as that. Even if you sometimes don't feel like you're receiving it from others, you can always count on yourself.

Kindness is integral to your wellness journey. When you treat yourself with kindness, you acknowledge your worth, feel strengthened and motivated, and prioritize the things that'll support your health.

One way you can lead with kindness is by practising positive self-talk; the most influential and important conversations you have are the ones you have with yourself. When your inner voice is kind and encouraging, you can channel this inspired energy into your life. For example:

> I feel strong.
> I trust myself.
> I am capable.
> I can do this.
> I will succeed.

Your internal monologue should not be critical, exercise should not be a punishment and your "off" days do not define you. You achieve the best outcomes by being your biggest cheerleader.

STRONG

IS A STATE

OF MIND

STRENGTH TRAINING MYTHS

Myths to put women off training have existed since the creation of sport, with females frequently told that their bodies are fragile and unable to cope with physical activity. In the early twentieth century, male educators stated that the ideal female body was a slim one, starting a cultural shift that continues to cause anxiety around appearance today.

With the rise of female strength training, there's also been an increase in fitness fearmongering, with misinformation causing women to avoid exercise. Let's unpack these misconceptions:

- *"Strength training will make you look masculine/ bulky."*

  A muscular physique is not a masculine one, and the particular training regime we choose will contribute to the shape we develop. Putting on muscular "bulk" takes targeted practice, consistent effort and years of training. It won't happen accidentally or overnight. Besides, growth is not something to fear; strong female bodies are valid.

- *"You can spot reduce body fat."*

  We can't "tone" a specific body part. We can train

a particular muscle group (see page 47), but we can't shrink an isolated place.

- *"Soreness is a sign of a good workout."*

    While delayed onset muscle soreness (DOMS) shows we had an intense session and challenged our bodies, achiness isn't a measure of how effective a workout is. Not all sessions will leave us with DOMS, but that doesn't mean we weren't working hard or won't see progress.

- *"Time off will undo your hard work."*

    Our bodies need time to rest and recover, and days off allow our muscles to grow. Progress won't be undone after a week off, and even with more time out we'll retain our familiarity with exercises and form (see page 69). It takes about three weeks off from training to notice any difference in strength.

- *"Not everyone's built for strength training."*

    Everyone has the capacity for strength training. While women naturally have stronger legs, we're also able to develop enormous strength in our upper bodies. There are no rules about who can be strong.

Celebrating Your Journey

As you enter your strong woman era, it's important to remember that your approach will be unique. All journeys are different, but they're all worth celebrating.

When it comes to exercise, we already understand the impact of genetic potential. Beyond this, factors such as your current fitness level, relationship with exercise and health history will also influence your approach. You'll have personal preferences when it comes to wellness practices, your own mental, physical and emotional capacities, and individual goals (see pages 52–53).

Another thing to consider is your lifestyle; your time is ruled by schedules and commitments and only you can understand the unique demands of your life. You determine what it means to discover your strength because it's completely personal to you.

Your wellness journey will also have its own pace, often following a non-linear path with progress being made in its own time. There's nowhere you need to be already, you're not behind and there's no rush. Quick transformations and committed bursts won't bring long-lasting happiness; the key is developing sustainable habits that allow you to lead a healthy, fulfilling life. It's helpful to think about this journey as one that'll span your lifetime, incorporating daily practices into your routine so you can become your strongest self.

The final step to discovering your strength is remembering that fitness is not *that* serious. For many of us, we're fortunate enough that it's not a case of life and death, we're not professional athletes and this won't affect our livelihoods. Working out is not supposed to be stressful, and you can prioritize moving daily, fuelling your body and nurturing your headspace without it being all-consuming. Having fun and feeling joyful is part of it.

However you decide to approach your health, there's space for it within the strong community. You can be proud of yourself just for deciding to embark on this journey.

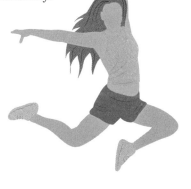

STRONGER THAN YOU KNOW

Women can sometimes doubt their strength, overlook their worth or limit themselves to "smaller" lives. As you look to start your strength training journey, it's essential that you remind yourself just how capable you are. It's up to you to acknowledge the depths of your strength and honour your power.

You can navigate uncomfortable feelings and experiences, handle pressure, take risks and brave the unknown. There's no challenge you cannot face or weight you cannot bear. In fact, data collected in 2023 found that women lift on average 1,556 kg (3,431 lb) per workout. Our minds and bodies are formidable, resilient and fierce.

It's important to recognize that you also have an enormous capacity for love, joy and happiness. You can hold both light and heavy emotions, overcome obstacles and accomplish great feats. Your life can be filled with positivity, growth and success.

You are stronger than you know – and it's time to get to know exactly what that means.

*The world
needs strong
women.*

AMY TENNEY

Entering Your Strong Woman Era

Let's take those first strides towards becoming strong together. We know we already possess the power – now's the time to take action, advocate for our own wellness and set ourselves on the path for success. As we enter this new phase of our lives, we can lead with the knowledge we've learned, the confidence we've developed and the strength we've grown.

Starting this journey can feel challenging, but we have to trust that we've got this: we are capable, we are courageous and we are ready to embrace this lifestyle.

This chapter will take you through tips that'll help you lead your strongest life by understanding your body, setting goals and creating a training programme. You will also discover techniques to boost your mental strength, such as being your own cheerleader, setting boundaries and reframing failures. As we'll cover in the following pages, it's important to remember that your approach will be unique, everyone's progress will look different and your support network will be on your side.

This next part is all about how we get strong.

YOUR VESSEL FOR STRENGTH

As you prepare yourself to start this strength training journey, let's first take a moment to discover more about your body, your vessel for strength. We should also consider your brain, the home of your thoughts and feelings.

When you feel stressed, your body tenses, your breathing quickens and your heart rate increases. When you exercise, your brain releases endorphins, dopamine and serotonin, relieving stress, raising motivation and elevating your mood. By acknowledging this mind–body connection, you can effectively identify your needs.

Brain

The cerebrum, the largest part of the brain, is split into two hemispheres, and each hemisphere has four lobes: frontal, parietal, temporal and occipital. When you exercise, the hippocampus (within the temporal lobe) is affected. This is the area of the brain responsible for learning, memories, processing and regulating emotions, language and aspects of visual perception. The temporal lobe is also the area responsible for your stress response.

Studies show training increases the number of blood vessels in and the volume of the hippocampus, which results in better circulation. This enables your organs to function optimally, your wounds to heal faster, your immune system to excel and your brain to operate at a greater capacity. Exercising also improves memory, helps you navigate your feelings and enhances cognitive function.

Body

There are more than 650 skeletal muscles in the body. The frontal lobe of the brain enables the precise and voluntary movements of these muscles. The skeletal muscles that are relevant to strength training fit into six major muscle groups. To optimize your workouts, you can programme routines around them (see pages 72–73).

Shoulders: Front, side and rear deltoids.
Arms: Biceps and triceps.
Chest: Pectorals.
Back: Latissimus dorsi, trapezius and rhomboids.
Abdominals: Rectus abdominis, transverse abdominis and obliques. Your "core" is your entire midsection, including your abdominals, back muscles and muscles around the pelvis.
Legs: Quadriceps, hamstrings, adductors, abductors, gluteal muscles (gluteus maximus, medius and minimus) and calves.

This journey is your own; only you can control where you end up

Posture

Posture is important for everyday life – from improving movement to avoiding muscle tension – and ensures good form while strength training. It can even influence our mindset. In psychology, this body-influencing-brain phenomenon is called embodied cognition.

Training our eyeline upwards and raising our heads slightly can instantly boost our mood because this posture helps us channel an uplifted feeling. Similarly, standing in a "power pose" in the gym can alleviate feelings of anxiety.

The general rule for good posture – something that is essential for safe strength training – is to imagine you're being pulled upwards by a golden thread attached to your head. While doing this, roll your shoulders back and down, think about connecting your ribs to your pelvis and soften your knees.

PERSONALIZING YOUR APPROACH

There are several factors to consider when starting strength training, and these can help you decide your approach. By assessing your options and understanding your motivations, you can build the foundations of tailored, fulfilling and long-lasting routines.

Your "Why"

Your "why" is your drive. Why strength training, why now, why you? Answer these questions to inform your practice:

How would you describe your current relationship with exercise?

What have your previous experiences with exercise been like?

What have or haven't you enjoyed before? What do you think you might enjoy?

What has made you consider strength training?

What excites you about strength training? Does anything intimidate you?

Why will you commit to pursuing strength training?

When it comes to the practice of strength training, consider the following:

- Where you train
- When you train
- Who you train with
- How long you train for
- How many times a week you train
- What muscle groups you target
- What exercises you complete
- What equipment you use

Once you acknowledge how you intend to approach strength training, you can start setting goals to align with your practice. Always remember that strength is personal. Entering your strong woman era means doing strong your way.

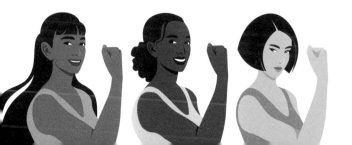

Setting Goals

Goals help shape and define our wellness journeys. They guide our practice, focus our minds and allow us to keep track of our progress along the way. Setting, sticking with and achieving our goals takes its own kind of strength.

When it comes to setting goals, bear the **SMART** acronym in mind: ensure your goals are **S**pecific, **M**easurable, **A**chievable, **R**elevant and **T**ime-bound. Consider all aspects of your health, thinking back to the eight dimensions of wellness. The aim is to give your energy to things that will improve your overall well-being.

Don't underestimate yourself! It's important to set short- and long-term goals that vary in difficulty. Having a handful of quick-win goals can help you feel a sense of achievement sooner and inspire you to keep going. More challenging goals will act as a framework for your journey, and they are incredibly fulfilling when met.

SMART short-term goals might be to join a gym, invest in some protein powder, create a wellness ritual or learn a specific exercise by the end of the month. You could also arrange a time to see a friend before the weekend to elevate your mood, or boost your strength training knowledge by reading this book before you start your training programme.

SMART long-term goals might include being able to lift a certain weight, feeling confident enough to wear a particular outfit, prepping a fixed number of meals in advance every week, sticking to a specific training programme for a length of time or regularly completing some of the wellness practices detailed across these pages.

You can create goals in isolation or you can plot a path from one achievement to the next. By breaking a goal down into smaller steps, you can map your success and celebrate every feat of strength.

The most rewarding goals will be personal to you and your journey. Their purpose is to motivate and steer you, and they can be adapted to reflect the evolving relationship you have with yourself and your attitude towards your health. Write your goals down and refer to them whenever you need to keep you on track.

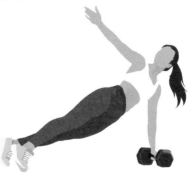

YOUR STRENGTH ROUTINE

"How do I actually start?" That's the question lots of us have when we first consider strength training. It's important to remember that you don't need to know everything (and no one actually does!). To start, you can hone a few exercises, grow more confident using weights and follow a simple routine.

- **The exercises:** Select a handful of exercises you are familiar with or that you'd like to learn and practise these. (See pages 130–151 for a selection.) You probably already know more than you think; your body naturally completes certain movements during daily life, such as squats when you sit down.

  Picking three to six exercises that target your full body (i.e. working across the muscle groups mentioned on pages 46–47) helps you develop all-round strength and build a powerful foundation for your fitness journey.

- **The weight:** You could choose to complete solely bodyweight exercises, movements using free weights, or a combination of both. All of these options will help you increase mobility, learn form and grow strength.

If you're using free weights, such as dumbbells, practise the exercise with a few different weights, starting "light" and judging how it feels. Work out which weight you can complete 8–12 repetitions of the exercise with. If you're able to complete 12 reps with ease, the weight is too light. You can progress your training by incrementally increasing the reps or weight.

Aim to complete 8–12 reps of each exercise. Each of these 8–12 reps is called a set. Practise 3–4 sets of each exercise, with 1-minute rests between them. This will mean you're doing your three to six exercises 3–4 times over, for 8–12 reps each.

- **The routine:** You could stick with one routine every session, or you could create a couple of routines and alternate between them. Follow this programme for four to six weeks before changing it to ensure you make consistent progress without plateauing.

A girl should
be two things:
who and what
she wants.

COCO CHANEL

Daily Stretch

We can complete 5–10 minutes of stretching every day to relieve stress, aid recovery and increase our range of motion (ROM). Strength and flexibility go hand in hand, so training one can improve the other.

Try this full-body flow:

1 **Deep Lunge:** Sink into a deep lunge, resting your back leg on the floor. You could take both arms up or one over towards the knee.

2 **Extended Child's Pose:** Sit back on your heels. Reach forwards until your forehead touches the floor, then reach to the left and right.

3 **Downward-Facing Dog Pose:** Rock your weight over your hands, tuck your toes and send your hips towards the ceiling. You could alternate touching your heels to the floor or extend each leg one at a time.

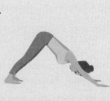

GROWING CONFIDENCE

Confidence and strength are closely related. When we feel confident, we're more able to do what we want, say what we mean and present the strongest versions of ourselves. When we feel strong, we tend to feel more confident. In fact, research shows that women feel 48 per cent more confident and 52 per cent happier when exercising regularly. But it's not always easy.

Many women struggle with confidence. A recent study on the gender exercise gap reveals 55 per cent of women report low self-confidence as a barrier to training, 58 per cent don't feel sporty enough to participate and only 11 per cent feel "very confident" exercising in public. This sense of imposter syndrome and concern over how we're perceived can prevent us from prioritizing our health.

Confident Woman Era

Confidence affects people of all ages, at different stages of their lives, across the world. Female confidence is often regarded as a societal issue where showing strength and leadership can be dubbed "masculine". The confidence gap means many women feel less inclined to prioritize themselves. We self-reject, modify our behaviour and inadvertently limit ourselves. When we close this space and embrace our strength, we can achieve anything we put our minds to.

Just like strength, we can grow our confidence through internal and external practices, such as:

- Challenging negative beliefs and feelings of self-doubt.

- Surrounding ourselves with supportive people.

- Acknowledging positive things about ourselves.

- Practising being present and assertive.

- Celebrating our wins and avoiding comparisons.

- Doing things we're good at and reminding ourselves of our value.

- Practising self-care and affirmations.

- Honouring our voice, practising confident posture and body language, and saying "No".

- Setting ourselves challenges.

- Embracing a growth mindset and championing our success.

Setting Yourself Up for Success

Your strength routine is the first step to training success. Beyond creating and following a programme, there are other things you can do both inside and outside the gym to maximize your results.

Inside the Gym

- **Wear suitable clothing:** Dress in sportswear you can move and feel comfortable in. For strength training, wear trainers with a flat sole (i.e. no platform or cushioning) or weightlifting shoes.

- **Complete an effective warm-up and cool-down:** See pages 70–71.

- **Use assists:** Chalk helps you grip the weights, plates under your heels aid squat form, using a bench or box for push-ups (see page 143) reduces the load going through your arms, and resistance bands offset your bodyweight while performing pull-ups (see page 137). In the future, you may consider using weightlifting straps for grip, weightlifting wraps or a belt for stability, and weightlifting sleeves for mobility.

- **Match your music:** Find playlists that match the beats per minute (BPM) of your workout heart rate.

- **Hydrate:** Drink water before, during and after your session. If you're training for longer than an hour, consider consuming a sports drink with electrolytes.
- **Breathe:** Breathe out with the "effort" or practise the Valsalva manoeuvre (see page 23).

Outside the Gym

- **Stock a gym bag:** Consider which items support your training, e.g. a glute band for warming up, a barbell pad for cushioning the bar, a water bottle and headphones.
- **Fuel your body:** Eat a balanced and nutritious diet. To build muscle, consume 1.6–2.2 grams of protein per kilogram of bodyweight. In the future, you may consider supplements (see page 99).
- **Practise mobility:** Follow online mobility routines to improve your range of motion.
- **Schedule rest days:** Allow your body time off to recover between sessions (see pages 84–85).
- **Create pre- and post-workout rituals:** See page 87.
- **Grow your knowledge:** Discover more about the areas you're interested in – starting with this book! Use this information to enhance your sessions.

PERMIT

YOURSELF

TO LIVE

POWERFULLY

Building Your Support Network

You don't have to do anything alone; you can build a support network. Knowing when to ask for help takes incredible self-awareness and strength.

- **General support:** Turn to your family, friends or partner for all-round support. You might discover you have people around you who are following similar paths, who you can share knowledge and motivation with. Take the time to explain what it is you're doing, express your feelings and share your progress.

- **General guidance:** The internet can be a useful source of information for how to complete specific exercises, examples of training routines and general wellness advice.

- **Personalized guidance:** A personal trainer is qualified to create tailored workout routines and provide 1:1 instruction. While nutritionists can offer general nutritional advice, in the UK only dietitians are qualified to provide diet and meal plans. Wellness coaches address your lifestyle and general well-being.

- **Health support:** Always consult a medical professional about any health concerns you may have.

STRONGER TOGETHER

We're surrounded by strong women who are authentically themselves, pursuing their passions and living their best lives. In sport, we can look to the likes of Billie Jean King, Junko Tabei, Florence Griffith Joyner, Simone Biles and Ilona Maher. In our own circles, we can think about people we respect and admire. We can take inspiration from each other, and find motivation and celebrate our strength together.

Women support women by being kind, building relationships and acknowledging each other's successes. Showing respect, giving praise, helping each other out, being on side and talking each other up can have a huge impact.

It's important to remember that we can succeed together; we have the strength to lift each other up. There's no comparison or competition – someone else's progress doesn't take away from our own – and there's space for all of us to thrive. Be supportive of others and surround yourself with people who support you. When women collaborate, we discover just how strong we are.

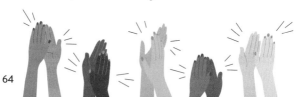

Every woman's
success should
be an inspiration
to another.
We're strongest
when we cheer
each other on.

SERENA WILLIAMS

Being Your Own Cheerleader

We spend a lot of time in our own heads. Most of us have an internal monologue that runs ten times faster than verbal speech, expressing our thoughts, feelings and intuition. It's a voice we hear constantly, and we can use this to strengthen our minds, bodies and spirits.

"Being your own cheerleader" means being on your own side. By recognizing your growth, praising your efforts and celebrating your wins, you instil a sense of self-belief and self-respect, and increase your chance of success. In fact, studies show that positive self-talk improves athletic performance and focus. You can control the narrative you hear daily, using this influence to motivate and inspire you. Remember how powerful your voice is.

You understand yourself best, so you can hone your ability to identify what you need from your inner cheerleader: encouragement, approval, sympathy or strength.

Measuring Progress

Just as we can find power in our voices, we can also take strength from our actions. Pursuing our own progress can be incredibly motivating. When we take steps towards where we want to be, we assert control over our well-being and champion our success. To be able to recognize when progress has been made, we need to determine what progress means to us.

Progress is defined as onwards movement; when we think about progress, we often think about achievement. The truth is, we don't need to be constantly on the up or ticking off accomplishments to be making progress.

There's strength in consistency, in commitment and in showing up and simply trying. While mindset shifts and physical feats might make for more measurable progress, we can't overlook the value of the "smaller" steps. When we view every action as positive momentum, we recognize that we can never undo progress, but rather learn from the process.

THE STRENGTH SPECTRUM

We know that being strong looks, feels and simply *is* different for everyone – it's relative and personal. Beyond our emotional, intellectual and spiritual strength (among the other dimensions), there are specific types of physical strength we can practise through training:

- **Strength endurance:** Your ability to perform repetitions of an exercise for an extended period of time, e.g. squats for 12–20 reps.

- **Explosive strength:** Your ability to use your strength at speed, e.g. box jumps.

- **Agile strength:** Your ability to control weight across multiple planes, e.g. lateral jumps.

- **Maximum strength:** Your ability to lift your maximum weight for a single repetition of an exercise, e.g. one-rep max (1RM) deadlift.

- **Static strength:** Your ability to hold a position where the muscles are contracted and there's an increase in tension, e.g. plank (see page 148).

- **Grip strength:** Your ability to hold onto objects, e.g. dead hang (see page 137).

STRONG FORM

When it comes to the practice of strength training, maintaining form optimizes our efforts, meaning we target the intended muscles, protect ourselves from injury and adopt effective technique. These general cues are helpful to remember:

- **Keep your head in line with your spine:** Don't crane your neck or tuck your chin. (Exceptions to the latter include hip thrusts – see page 135 – and crunches – see page 149.) Allow your head to travel with your spine.

- **Don't lock out:** "Locking out" means excessively extending your joints. Keep your elbows and knees "soft" (slightly bent) during exercise.

- **Engage your core:** Your core is a huge source of strength and stability. Brace the muscles in your middle and maintain this internal pressure while lifting.

- **Drive:** Keep the tension through your muscles as you move the weight. Channel effort through your contact points, such as your feet on the floor.

- **Breathe:** Don't forget to breathe! Inhale and exhale with intention.

WARMING UP AND COOLING DOWN

Warming up before exercising helps prepare the body for movement and avoid injury, pumping oxygen into the muscles, loosening our joints and increasing our flexibility. It's also essential to cool down after a workout to allow the heart rate to decrease, the body to recover and the muscles to stretch out.

	Warm-up	Cool-down
Type	Dynamic stretches (moving stretches)	Static stretches (holding stretches) or developmental stretches (deeper stretches to improve your flexibility)
Exercises include	Arm circles, leg swings, hip circles, squat-to-reach	Overhead triceps stretch, standing hamstring stretch, butterfly pose, cobra pose

	Warm-up	Cool-down
Reps/Time	10 reps of each	15–30 seconds of each
Equipment	Bodyweight, resistance bands, glute band	Bodyweight, resistance bands, foam roller

Both warm-ups and cool-downs should focus on the muscle group you're training or have trained. They should last around 10 minutes and largely use your bodyweight.

What About Cardio?

If strength is your focus, complete cardiovascular activity after lifting weights. This'll prevent pre-workout fatigue, ensure that you're primed to build more muscle (because the muscle-building enzymes are more effective when resistance training comes first) and help you lift heavier. Some research shows that you'd ideally separate strength training and cardio by at least 6 hours to see improvements with both – but this depends on your goals.

To get the most out of your efforts, prioritize the movement that's most important to you and practise a structured routine that includes an effective warm-up and cool-down.

CREATING A PROGRAMME

To grow stronger with training, we can follow a programme. A strength training programme is a set of structured routines we practise for a four-to-six-week block, tracking the exercises we complete, the weights we use and the sets and reps we perform. By recording these details, we can ensure we make consistent progress as we maintain or increase the weight, sets or reps every week.

While we can choose to change our workouts every session, sticking with a programme for the duration of the training block focuses our efforts on growth. We can keep track of our programme by using phone notes, an app or a notepad.

- **The split:** Consider how you'd like to separate the exercises you want to complete over the course of a week. You can "split" your sessions however you like, such as by having upper body and lower body days, grouping together push movements, pull movements and leg exercises, or by focusing on each muscle group in turn. Alternatively, you could continue to practise full-body workouts.

  Ideally, you should leave 48 hours between training the same muscle group. For example, you'd have more effective workouts targeting your legs if you were to schedule them at least a couple of days apart.

- **The exercises:** Allocate three to six exercises to each of your routines. Compound movements are those that target multiple muscles; for example, a squat (a compound leg exercise) works your hamstrings, glutes, quadriceps, calves and core. Accessory exercises isolate one muscle; for example, a calf raise (an accessory leg exercise) works your calves. When planning your routines, include a mixture of compound and accessory movements, starting each session with your compound lifts.

- **The equipment:** Free weights and machines (see pages 128–129) work many of the same muscles. While machines only allow you to move within a fixed range of motion, free weights allow for more creativity. You can typically lift more weight with machines, but free weight exercises can be highly effective because they work more muscles. Try to include a combination of both in your programme.

Checking In

As we continue with our wellness journeys it's important that we regularly check in with ourselves and review our thoughts, feelings, actions and behaviours. By allowing ourselves the space to assess how we're doing, we connect with our emotions, grow our self-awareness and develop our mental strength.

It's up to us to decide what these check-ins look like, how long they last and how often we complete them. We might conduct internal reviews, keep a journal, or discuss our thoughts with our support networks. With strength training, we might reflect at the ends of our sessions or after each training block. What matters most is that we permit ourselves the time and energy to process how we're getting on and plot a path forwards.

Ask yourself:
What am I thinking right now?
How am I feeling right now?
What actions am I taking right now?
What behaviours am I practising right now?
How am I channelling my strength right now?

Mental Strength Training

Just as we can follow specific training routines and schedule in workouts, it's important we also find time to engage with targeted mental health practices. Both mental and physical health exercises are essential to our well-being and can boost our confidence, help us grow and make us feel strong.

Mental strength training includes developing coping strategies for dealing with uncomfortable feelings, honing relaxation techniques and allowing ourselves the space to acknowledge and express our emotions. We can support our mental resilience by practising positive thinking patterns, learning to accept change, building connections with others and facing our fears. As with strength training, we'll see more progress if we follow routines, complete regular check-ins and are responsive to our needs.

We already understand the relationship between the different areas of strength; working on one positively impacts the others. By dedicating time to both our mental and physical wellness, we empower ourselves to lead all-round stronger lives.

Setting Boundaries

The idea of women reclaiming and redefining "strong" won't appeal to everyone. While *we* get it, some people simply won't understand. It's important to remember that it's not our responsibility to convince others of the value of what we're doing, but it can be useful to consider how we can navigate misconceptions, unsolicited advice and criticism.

When it comes to the how, what and why of strength training, some people will apply their own stereotypes and biases. They might misconstrue our motivation, misinterpret our goals or undermine our efforts. When faced with judgement like this, know that there isn't any wisdom to be gleaned from someone else's negativity and we don't need to be affected by it. They don't get it, and that's on them.

Other people might feel the need to give unsolicited advice. While we can appreciate guidance when we have asked for it, unsolicited advice is often someone else inserting themselves into a situation. This person won't know what it is we're trying to do or why we're doing it, but they'll tell us what they think anyway. Unsolicited advice can be extremely off-putting and unhelpful, so we don't have to take it on board.

We may also experience criticism from people who are intimidated by our strength and feel insecure about their own. These individuals are often on destructive paths, and we can't allow them to interfere with our journeys. The best thing we can do is distance ourselves from these people and block the toxicity.

Ultimately, we navigate these situations by setting boundaries. We can determine what we expect from others and refuse to settle for less. By valuing our headspace and advocating for our own journeys, we strengthen our commitment to ourselves and the strong woman era.

Gym Etiquette

These are some unspoken rules all gym-goers should follow (in no particular order):

1 Don't give unsolicited advice.
2 Be mindful of your surroundings.
3 Avoid "hoarding" equipment.
4 Clean your weights.
5 Put your equipment back.

Life's obstacles seem lighter when you feel strong enough to lift them

FACTORS THAT INFLUENCE STRENGTH

Strength fluctuates – we always possess it, but how strong we feel changes. Understanding the factors that influence strength can help us support our growth.

- **Food:** Fuelling our bodies is essential for daily function and strength. We should prioritize nutritious, protein-rich meals, wholegrain carbohydrates, healthy fats and lots of fruit and vegetables.

- **Fluids:** We need to drink enough water for both our brains and bodies. When we're dehydrated, our muscles cramp, our blood pressure drops and our mood falls.

- **Rest:** Getting adequate rest improves our focus, boosts our mood and helps us feel stronger.

- **Injuries:** Aches, twinges and injuries can impact our performance. We also feel weaker when we're unwell. Rest, gentle movement and rehabilitation exercises can help.

- **Hormones:** Oestrogen impacts our mood, energy and strength. Depending on where we are in our cycles, how strong we feel fluctuates (see pages 80–81). Stress hormones can break down and destroy muscle proteins, decreasing physical strength.

YOUR STRENGTH CYCLE

Your body goes through natural cycles every month and over the years, and these phases can affect your health. One series of hormonal changes you might experience is the menstrual cycle.

When you're on your period, your body might look and feel different. By acknowledging what your body is experiencing and adapting to its needs, you can continue to grow.

The follicular phase: The follicular phase starts on the first day of your period and lasts 10–14 days. While you may feel achy, tired and irritable during menstruation, your energy levels peak shortly after this time. Oestrogen and progesterone begin to rise, leaving you feeling livelier, happier and stronger.

Studies show that the menstrual cycle has no direct impact on muscular performance, but the effects of the hormones released during this phase can make you feel better in yourself and enable you to access greater mental and physical strength. This is the time of month to be productive, socialize with friends and focus on consistency with your training routine.

The ovulation phase: The ovulation phase occurs around day 14 of the menstrual cycle and lasts for 24 hours, although the high hormone levels can continue for three to four days (from the day the egg is released). Oestrogen and testosterone peak, resulting in increased confidence, extroversion and bravery. You can also feel more adventurous, have a higher pain threshold and experience an increased sex drive.

During this phase you might decide to push yourself more, try new things and strive towards your goals.

The luteal phase: The luteal phase takes place between days 15 and 28. Initially, progesterone rises, making you feel slower and more anxious. You can also experience bouts of sadness, bloating and a desire for comfort from food, activities and those around you. During the final days of your cycle, oestrogen and progesterone plunge, often resulting in low mood.

This is the time of month to take a gentler approach. You should prioritize self-care and be especially sensitive to your needs. On some days, rest might be the best thing. On others, movement can help you feel brighter.

FAILING STRONG

We can choose to view failure as a sign of weakness, or we can recognize it as an opportunity for growth.

Failure is never a step back, an indication of inadequacy or an invitation to quit. We build resilience, improve our focus and learn more about ourselves when things go "wrong".

When it comes to wellness, we might think of failure as falling out of our routine, struggling to stay motivated or not finding the same success from our usual practices. It can be useful to determine what we consider to be "failures" – without holding ourselves to unattainable standards. It's important that we regularly acknowledge all we've achieved and remind ourselves of our perseverance.

Training to Failure

"Training to failure" means completing as many repetitions of an exercise as we can until we physically can't do any more. It's about pushing ourselves to our limits and increasing the size and strength of our muscles. Although it can be challenging, "failure" is where growth happens.

Champions keep playing until they get it right.

BILLIE JEAN KING

Taking Rest Days

Rest is essential for our health and happiness. We can't always be "on", and we need to schedule downtime and rest days alongside our training routines and other commitments. When we take time out and commit to rest and recovery, we strengthen our minds and bodies.

Rest improves our mental strength by allowing our minds to clear, our thoughts to pause and our feelings to settle. By shifting the focus away from our worries, we can take a weight off and unwind. Then, when we feel able, we can return to the tasks at hand with rejuvenated energy.

For our bodies, the strength we build through rest is literal. When we exercise, we create small tears in the muscle fibres – and this can create DOMS. The body then rebuilds the damaged muscles bigger and stronger. For this process to occur effectively, we need to rest. Not only should we plan our sessions to accommodate 48 hours between training the same muscle groups so that the muscles can heal, we should also respond to how our bodies feel on a day-to-day basis.

As we continue to grow stronger, we'll learn to identify when we need rest and what approach would best serve us in that moment. There are two main forms of rest: active recovery and total rest days.

Active recovery: This involves non-strenuous activity to help our muscles recover. We might take this approach on the days between workouts. We could consider:

- Walking
- Light jogging
- Cycling
- Swimming
- Yoga
- Mobility
- Stretching
- Foam rolling

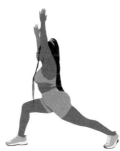

Total rest days: This involves complete rest to allow our bodies to relax. We might prefer this approach when we're feeling particularly drained. We could consider:

- Journalling
- Reading
- Colouring
- Listening to music
- Watching a film
- Meditating
- Having a hot bath
- Getting a massage

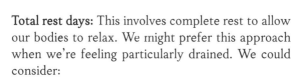

Meditation

Meditation and strength training naturally complement each other because both practices focus our minds and connect us with our bodies. While lifting weights is about power and movement, meditation is about being still: steadying our heart rate, reducing cortisol levels and helping us get more restorative rest.

We can practise meditation as part of our strength training routines, completing 5 minutes before working out, for example. This can help prepare our minds, relieve tension from our muscles and enable us to exert greater control over our bodies when exercising.

Try this meditation practice:

1 Find a comfortable, seated position.
2 Inhale deeply, allowing the oxygen to travel around your body. As you exhale, release any tension from your muscles.
3 With every deep breath, feel your motivation, energy and power grow. Invite strength to fill your body.

Daily Strength Rituals

A ritual is a series of actions we follow that adds structure and intention to our time. By practising these routines we support our total wellness, take steps towards our goals and create the foundations of a strong lifestyle. When it comes to creating daily rituals, it's helpful to consider what their purpose might be, how many stages would be involved and when we would complete them. These are some routines you could incorporate into your daily life:

Morning Ritual
1 Practise 5–10 minutes of meditation.
2 Complete a simple stretching routine.
3 Set your daily intentions.

Pre-Work or Pre-Study Ritual
1 Spend 5–10 minutes deep breathing outside.
2 Listen to your favourite song.
3 Complete a 5-minute hand massage.

Post-Gym Ritual
1 Wash your face and have a shower.
2 Empty and repack your gym bag.
3 Complete a post-workout check-in.

Reset Ritual
1 Clean and organize your space.
2 Write a new to-do list.
3 Practise 5–10 minutes of self-care.

Evening Ritual
1 Spend 5–10 minutes journalling.
2 Prepare any items you need for the next day.
3 Watch the sunset.

Committing to the Lifestyle

Now to commit. We know we have the strength and we understand how to access it – next we make this our lifestyle. By committing to the mindset, refining our approach and making a strong routine, we can continue to progress with our journeys for life.

This we know to be a worthy cause; our health and happiness are lifelong pursuits and deserve our continued investment. As we embrace our strong woman era, growth, passion and power become central to who we are. We can lead joyful and fulfilling lives where being in control, achieving our goals and prioritizing our well-being are priorities.

But committing can be hard; to make strong stick, it has to be sustainable. This chapter will keep you on the right path. From finding balance and creating habits to taking time off and optimizing your future, these pages will make being strong your new way of life. It's about being adaptable, advancing your routines and supporting your mental and physical growth.

As you commit to this lifestyle, strong becomes second nature. You dictate your own journey, and it's within your power to make this one last.

FINDING BALANCE

To commit to this lifestyle and make being strong sustainable, we need to have balance. We know wellness extends beyond exercise and, by balancing our responsibilities, we can take ownership of our time and create lasting routines.

Firstly, we need to consider what things we'd like to fit into our everyday lives. There are many demands of our time, including fixed commitments such as work, study and childcare, but we do have some flexibility with the remaining moments. It can be challenging to balance work, gym and errands with socializing, trips out and self-care. We can only juggle so much, so it's important that we prioritize the things that best support our health and happiness.

Being disciplined with fundamentals, like work and training, is essential, but we also need to find time to switch off. For some, the preferred approach is 80:20 – this is where we follow a structured routine for 80 per cent of the time and, with the remaining 20, we're more relaxed. This way, we balance the "I have tos" with the "I want tos".

When true balance is achieved, everything will slot into our schedules under a framework of total wellness. It's important to remember that strength training is supposed to be a supplement to a healthy lifestyle, not constitute the entirety of one.

Without balance, we risk slipping into the "all or nothing" approach. This means we sometimes advance full pelt towards our goals and other times we're completely put off by the thought. The "all or nothing" approach is incredibly draining and often leads to a yo-yo relationship with our health. Being fully in and then fully out is a spurt of passion rather than a fulfilling, long-term commitment to ourselves.

There are practices we can incorporate into our days to boost our mental and physical strength but, to live strong, we have to embrace the rest of life too.

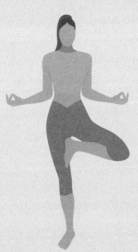

Daily Stability

Stability training requires balance, coordination and control. It improves our athletic performance and reduces our risk of injury. Practise these daily stability movements to connect you with your strength:

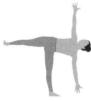

- **Hip Airplane:** Stand on one foot, spread your arms to Superwoman and tilt forwards, lifting your back leg. Then, rotate your hips away from your standing leg and open your chest to the side.

- **Bird Dog:** Start on your hands and knees. Point one arm out in front while extending your opposite leg behind you. Keep your core engaged and your arm, head, back and leg in a straight line.

- **Marching Glute Bridge:** Lie on your back with your knees bent, push through your heels and lift your pelvis. Alternate bringing a leg towards your chest.

A strong woman
knows she has
strength enough for
the journey, but a
woman of strength
knows it is in the
journey where she
will become strong.

ANONYMOUS

Creating Habits

We can choose to make wellness a habit by consistently dedicating time to our practice and working towards our goals. This means that "strong" becomes our routine. When motivation fails us, habit kicks in.

It takes a lot of discipline to keep showing up for ourselves, especially when the temptation is to return to old routines. To change this behaviour, we typically follow five stages:

1 **Precontemplation:** Unaware of need for change.

2 **Contemplation:** Acknowledgement of need for change.

3 **Preparation:** Planning to implement change.

4 **Action:** Making change.

5 **Maintenance:** Continuing change.

We could implement smaller practices or consider larger lifestyle changes, taking on each new habit one at a time. These changes could be broken down into smaller steps so that they feel more manageable. It's important that our habits honour our goals and support our total wellness. As we gradually enforce healthy habits, we form the foundations of a strong lifestyle.

SHOWING UP
AND STICKING
WITH IT TAKES
THE GREATEST
STRENGTH
OF ALL

BEING ACCOUNTABLE

We are in complete control of our wellness journeys. As we strive to make a long-term commitment to ourselves, it's important to remember that we are accountable for our choices. It's up to us whether we see this through, and we have to be open and honest with ourselves about our thoughts, feelings and behaviours.

We can break down our accountability into three parts: perseverance, acceptance and reflection.

1   **Perseverance:** We are accountable for our efforts, including those we don't expend. Perseverance in our wellness journeys means knowing when we can push through and choosing to do so. It means being so committed to our health and happiness that we honour our true limits, rather than self-rejecting or minimizing our power. With perseverance, we have the ability to distinguish between the challenging and the impossible. An example of this is working hard to get out those last reps of an exercise.

2   **Acceptance:** Acceptance comes after perseverance. This is when we know we've given all we can, and we appreciate this effort and respect our limits. Being accountable not only means being the

champions of our own success, but also being the protectors of our well-being; acknowledging that we've honoured our boundaries and celebrating that. An example of this is accepting that an imperfect meditation session is better than one you didn't do at all.

Remember, if you're operating at 40 per cent, putting in 40 is the same as you giving 100 per cent.

3 **Reflection:** By reflecting on our thoughts, feelings and behaviours, we take accountability for them, review how we're doing and improve our self-awareness. An example of this is journalling at the end of the day.

As much as we can hold ourselves accountable by recording and reflecting on our efforts, we can also enlist our support networks for help. We could share our intentions and ask our family and friends to check in on our progress, or we could see if they would accompany us as we complete one of our practices.

Investing in Wellness

Investing in our wellness is investing in our strong woman era. Deciding to dedicate time, energy and, on occasion, money to things that will boost our mood and enhance our strength indicates our commitment to our journeys.

We can, of course, make great progress without spending anything. We can practise bodyweight exercises at home, use free apps and write in old notebooks; "strong" has no price tag. But, while our health doesn't have to have any financial ties, it is incredibly valuable. As we continue to work towards our goals, we might decide to invest in our wellness.

Mental Health Investments

- **Journal:** Use a journal, diary or planner specifically for your wellness journey.
- **Toiletries:** Invest in skincare, bath products and essential oils to enhance self-care rituals. You might also consider candles, incense or a diffuser. Alternatively, you could experiment with making your own products.

- **Weighted blanket:** Relax with a weighted blanket to help you calm down and improve your sleep. You can also listen to soothing music or a guided meditation for free.

- **Books:** Buy reading, colouring or activity books to accompany wellness practices. Affirmation cards might also be a valuable investment, or you could create your own using page 15.

Physical Health Investments

- **Gym membership:** Try free day or class passes first, then sign up to a monthly membership. These vary in price but the same is true of all: the more often you go, the more you get for your money.

- **Home gym equipment:** At first you could look to get a lighter and heavier set of dumbbells, a couple of resistance bands and an exercise mat.

- **Supplements:** Depending on your goals, you might buy protein powder and a shaker. Creatine is another go-to supplement that improves muscular performance, strength and mass. You might also consider pre-workout powder for an endurance, energy and focus boost.

- **Training clothes:** Invest in outfits that allow you to move, stretch and sweat.

I love working with weights. I knew they'd give me the strength I needed.

FLORENCE GRIFFITH JOYNER

KEEPING FOCUS

Our commitment is to being strong and, as part of this, it's important that we're able to recognize when certain attitudes become unhealthy. There's a difference between being focused and being obsessed; we can be motivated without fuelling self-criticism, and we can collaborate with our bodies rather than punish them.

The question we need to ask is, *"How is this behaviour helping me achieve my goals?"* As we consider this, remember that this journey is intended to unite our strong minds, bodies and spirits. If we start to head in the opposite direction, it's likely our focus has shifted to something conflicting, unsustainable and potentially toxic.

Lost-focus red flags include feeling burned out, experiencing low mood and excusing unhealthy behaviours, such as undereating or overexercising. If we notice ourselves beginning to adopt a harmful mindset, it's vital that we take the time to stop what we're doing, check in with how we're feeling and make the necessary changes to ensure our focus remains on our health and happiness.

ADVANCING A PROGRAMME

As this new lifestyle becomes routine, we might decide to challenge ourselves by reconfiguring our sessions. We already know our training programmes should change every four to six weeks to maximize our progress, but how do we go about this?

- **Same goals; similar challenge:** If we're working towards the same goals, our programmes won't necessarily change much each training block. We'd likely keep the same weekly split and substitute a few of the exercises or change the order. It's normal to always perform staples (like squats, deadlifts and pull-ups) within our routines, so we might find we never remove certain lifts from our programmes.

- **Same goals; different challenge:** While our goals may be the same, after a few training blocks we might welcome different challenges. We could incorporate more unilateral (single-limb) exercises, pulses or pauses, or tempo work (adjusting the speed we complete each rep). Other challenges include supersets (completing two exercises one after the other), tri-sets (completing three exercises one after the other) and drop sets (lifting a weight until failure, immediately picking up a lighter weight and continuing until failure). We also might face new time constraints and need to adjust our split, combine sessions or condense our routines.

- **Different goals:** Our programmes change to reflect our goals. We might complete similar routines but work within different rep ranges. For example:

> To develop strength and power: 3–5 sets of 1–6 reps; to develop muscle: 3–4 sets of 8–12 reps; to develop muscular endurance: 2–3 sets of 12–20+ reps.

We could also look to incorporate other exercise disciplines, such as cardiovascular training.

It's important to remember that it's up to us how we choose to pursue our strength. Our focus should always be on our goals and the challenges we'd like to face. However we commit to this lifestyle, whether by following a structured programme or by having a more flexible routine, is valid. No one gets to gatekeep "strong".

Being Adaptable

While we can organize our time and structure our routines, one of the best skills we can hone throughout our journeys is adaptability. By being adaptable, we can stay on track to achieve our goals, even when plans change. This way, we never have to compromise on being strong.

We can be adaptable in a number of ways. For example, by changing the practices we choose to complete, being flexible with our time and adjusting our goals. With strength training, we can modify movements through regressions or progressions (decreasing or increasing the demands of movements), we can use different equipment and we can complete variations of exercises. By being open to adapting our routines, we limit the variables that might prevent us from committing to our strength.

It's helpful to have backup plans and variations of our routines ready for the busier periods of our lives. Equipped with options, we can adapt to our changing needs and continue to support our growth.

Changing Your Routine

The first routine you create is unlikely to suit you forever, especially as you experience different phases of your life. To make being strong sustainable, your routine has to change.

While you can adapt as you go, sometimes the best option is a fresh start. It's important to remember that there are no rules for when you pursue this new approach. It doesn't have to be centred around an event, wait until Monday or accompany the new year – you can change your routine as soon as you recognize it's no longer compatible with your life.

Rethinking your routine too often can make you feel unsettled and uncommitted, but knowing when it's time for something different enables you to continue working towards your goals. Your routine often needs to change when your life does, but you can choose to refresh it without the catalyst of a life event – for example, by prioritizing a new hobby, experimenting with different forms of movement or pursuing a unique set of goals.

OWNING YOUR STRENGTH

We know there are many ways we can practise being strong. As we commit to this lifestyle, it's essential we allow ourselves to own our strength.

It's easy to default to old behaviours, but you're entitled to be proud of who you are, welcome your growth and channel your full power. "Strong" translates into every area of your life and it's something you carry with you always: trusting in your ability, advocating for your well-being and pioneering your success. Strength training can help you feel this way, with a survey in 2023 showing that after a workout women feel accomplished, energized and unstoppable.

We know we *are* strong, so it's important we allow ourselves to *be* strong. Of course, it's nearly impossible to always feel this way, but we can return to "strong" as our state of being. Let's embrace this mindset as integral to who we are: strong women leading strong lives.

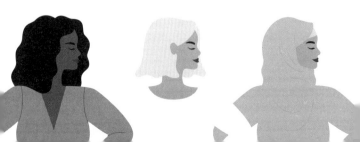

Strong is a collaboration of the mind, body and spirit

Mindfulness

Being mindful is a core component of supporting a strong headspace. Mindfulness is a practice that not only serves us in daily life, but also when strength training. By bringing our awareness to ourselves, our feelings and the present moment, we become grounded in our bodies. Mindfulness can help us overcome feelings of gym anxiety, find motivation and strengthen our mind–muscle connection (i.e. mentally recruiting the required muscles) – something that is essential for effective resistance training.

Practise connecting with your body as you embrace your strong woman era:

- **Muscle Mindfulness:** Without moving, try to tense and relax each of your muscles.

- **Hand Mindfulness:** Pressing your hands on a surface, focus your weight through your palms, then through your fingers.

- **Feet Mindfulness:** While standing, push all of your weight through your heels, then try spreading it through your toes.

TAKING TIME OFF

To make being strong sustainable, we need to allow ourselves time off. Working towards our goals is rewarding, but it can also lead to a build-up of fatigue. Being able to identify when we need time off enables us to take care of our mental and physical well-being and stay committed to our journeys.

Unlike scheduled rest days, time off means taking a break from our usual routines – for example, by taking a deload week (decreasing the intensity of our workouts). Remember, time off won't undo progress.

Feeling...

Sore: Take an impromptu rest day.

Fatigued/Like you've plateaued: Have a week off and prioritize rest. Or take a deload week to help your body recover and feel ready to get stronger the following week. You could also assess your routines.

Injured: Take as long off from your routines as required and focus on rehabilitation.

Overwhelmed: Stop everything and take some time to evaluate this feeling. When you feel ready, start afresh with new routines.

Unmotivated: Show up and see how you feel.

Growing with Your Body

Bodies change. They can fluctuate hourly, daily, yearly and over the course of your life – and it's something you never need to justify. You can't be limited to one shape or size forever; you have to allow yourself to grow. Decide what "growth" means to you and how you want to pursue it.

It's important to recognize mental and emotional growth as you commit to your journey, but you should also embrace physical changes, because they reflect your life and your experiences.

By being open to fluctuations in your appearance, you learn to value your body as it is and your happiness won't depend on the way you look. You will always exist within your body, so it's vital that you always show it love, care and respect. Your worth has nothing to do with your appearance.

Growth occurs in its own time. While you can facilitate physical changes through exercise, some things are beyond your control. Just as you look different now than you did when you were younger, you will see natural changes as you get older. You'll also notice differences in your appearance depending on the time of day, where you are in your menstrual cycle and what you've eaten. Your body can even take on other forms as you go through different life events and biological changes.

While bodies do change, they're not seasonal. You shouldn't forcibly cycle your body through gain and loss phases because this attitude can be unhealthy, unfulfilling and unsustainable. To grow with your body, you have to allow it the space to become what you're asking of it: strong enough to lift, powerful enough to move, fuelled enough to flourish, calm enough to breathe, happy enough to heal and celebrated enough to thrive.

How you look can change, but being strong is permanent. Let's continue to develop the relationship we have with ourselves and appreciate our bodies for being constant sources of strength in our lives.

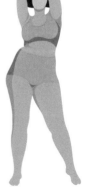

WEARING THE SHORTS

We are entitled to wear whatever we like, without having to "prepare" our bodies first. Clothes can impact our mood, communicate our personalities and help us feel more confident. There are no rules for what certain body types are allowed to wear – we can wear shorts, sports bras, bikinis or any other items of clothing.

The truth is that people make money selling insecurities. The myth about female body hair being unsightly and unhygienic came from razor manufacturers trying to expand their market in the early twentieth century. We've long been sold the idea that very natural and normal parts of the female form – body hair, cellulite, thread veins, stretch marks, hip dips, skin rolls – are unattractive and should be concealed, and now we're refusing to buy this narrative.

There's nothing "wrong" with the way we look, and we shouldn't feel shamed into limiting our wardrobes. The only step required for wearing shorts is to put them on. Remember, we change clothes to fit our bodies, not the other way around.

When
the world
tells you
to shrink,
expand.

ELAINE WELTEROTH

Defining Feminine

We are strong women, but sometimes we can find ourselves limited by a version of femininity that we've been taught. This ideal comes with its own appearance, attitude and traits, and "strong" often becomes highjacked.

As this lifestyle becomes routine, it's important to remember that we define feminine for ourselves. Strength training isn't about building a more "womanly" figure or allowing growth within the parameters of someone else's version of femininity. We decide how we feel our strongest and we choose to follow our own paths. How we look, how we feel and how we act are strong and feminine because these things coexist.

Feminine ideals include courage, creativity, empathy, passion, sensitivity and intuition – but we're also multifaceted and find that other behaviours align with our identities. We can find freedom in allowing ourselves to simply be and claiming "strong" for women. There isn't one way to exist powerfully and weight training can be whatever we make it. This is how women *do* strong.

WATCH HOW
MUCH YOU GROW,
CELEBRATE ALL
YOU BUILD, LIVE
THIS WAY FOR LIFE

STOPPING COMPARISONS

Comparison can be second nature to many of us; we look at others and feel that we have to or cannot compete. We see someone else's appearance, success or life and tell ourselves we should be more like them. These thoughts are often harmful occupiers of our headspace and mean that we overlook our innate value and unique journeys.

As we commit to the strong mindset, we can learn to become more aware of our thought patterns and challenge those that don't serve us. The truth about comparison is that we always see through our own lens of preference and bias, meaning we never really get the full story. It's incredibly unkind and unfair for us to hold ourselves to standards that don't exist.

For example, when we look at someone, we're only ever able to register how they look in that moment *to us*. Not how they looked after

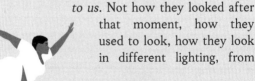

that moment, how they used to look, how they look in different lighting, from

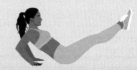

different angles, at different times of day, or to themselves. We don't know how they train or how long they have been training for, what their goals are and what progress they've made, or what their lifestyle and nutrition are like. We have no idea of their health history, their genetic potential, or the journey they're on. We're comparing our entire selves with a snippet, curated online or fleeting in real life, of someone else.

Looking at someone's physique, workout regime, diet or lifestyle and comparing our own means we lose perspective of our needs. We won't look like someone else by imitating their daily meals or following their strength training programmes because we are unique in everything that makes us up. How we do "strong" is completely valid.

It's important to recognize that women can win together. We're not in a competition, we're not the same and there's no judgement for how we approach this lifestyle.

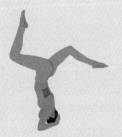
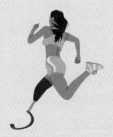

Living Strong

Strong is our present – we want to be our happiest, healthiest selves right now – but it's also important that we recognize strong is our future. By taking a proactive approach to our health, we can optimize our entire lives.

Active ageing means continuing to invest in the eight dimensions of wellness, including our emotional, physical and social wellness, over the course of our lives to extend healthy life expectancy. We all get older, and we can control part of what this will entail for us by investing in our well-being now. Through mental health practices, diet, strength training, aerobic activity (e.g. walking), flexibility exercises and social interactions, we can live healthier for longer.

There are some natural side effects of ageing, but we can continue to lead with the strong mindset for life. Remember that getting older is a privilege and be grateful to your mind and body for accompanying you on this journey. Ultimately, being strong is a commitment that spans our lifetimes, offering payoffs forever.

SETTING LIFE GOALS

By this point we understand how strength impacts every area of our lives. Feeling mentally and physically strong helps us accomplish great feats and fortify our own paths. As our strength develops, our expectations of what it's possible for us to achieve broaden. Emboldened by our capacity for growth and success, we can set life goals.

Different from our specific wellness goals (see pages 52–53), life goals encompass our entire lives and focus on long-term fulfilment. They might involve relationships, personal development, our careers or our homes. It can be helpful to look at our wider lives and establish what changes we'd like to see. We can be empowered by our strength progress and our ability to overcome, build and thrive.

It's important to take the time to consider your life goals and note them down somewhere you can be reminded of them often. These reminders can help you create and lead your strongest life.

Let's dream big, explore different avenues and be excited about all that's yet to come!

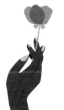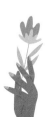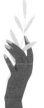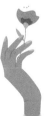

STRONG FOR GENERATIONS

As women who train, it's up to us to empower the next generation of strong girls. We can reshape the health and wellness industry and create a space that celebrates all bodies, abilities and forms of movement. "Strong" is something we've already claimed for ourselves; now it's time to show our sisters, nieces, daughters and friends what it means to run, throw and lift "like a girl".

By challenging negative messaging, breaking stereotypes and abandoning harmful fads, phrases and attitudes, we can foster a community that supports young women on their total wellness journeys. Health is not about appetite-suppressing lollipops, exercise trackers, or phrases like "Strong not skinny". So, let's build a safe space for women to discover their strength without pressure, judgement or criticism.

Through our influence online or in real life, we can encourage women to train, be strong and develop healthy relationships with themselves. By modelling ourselves as strong women leading strong lives, we inspire those around us to recognize their worth, prioritize their well-being and achieve their goals. Strength training is already becoming more normalized for women, and we can continue to reinforce this message by showing up and committing to our health.

From how we approach activity to the way we talk about our bodies, future strong women can adopt these behaviours and learn the new narrative: this *is* "strong". We have the power to uplift the younger generations with the strength we've discovered in ourselves.

And it's not just about encouraging young girls; strength has no age limit. We can empower our mothers, grandmothers and aunties to embrace their strength and live their best lives. These are the generations of the cabbage soup diet, leotards and the "If you can pinch more than an inch" mentality. They too deserve to enter this new age of female wellness, growth and strength.

This is not only our strong woman era – it's *the* strong woman era.

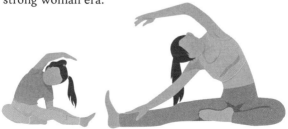

Conscious Movement

The form we adopt while strength training is often beneficial for day-to-day tasks. By being conscious of the way we move our bodies, we can call on the correct muscles, reduce our risk of injury and optimize activity. As we connect more with our bodies through exercise, we learn how to complete effective, daily functional movements.

It's likely we already perform these every day:

- **Squat** – sitting down on a chair.
- **Calf Raise** – tiptoeing to reach something up high.
- **Stiff-Leg Deadlift** – reaching with straight legs to pick something up off the floor (see page 134).
- **Front Raise** – lifting something out in front of you.
- **Farmer's Walk** – carrying items in your hands over a distance.

Say I am movement,
that I am the year,
and I am the era of
the women.

AMANDA GORMAN

Strength Training Fundamentals

It's time to get to work! Strength training is for everyone and, supported by the practical guidance in this chapter, you can commit to lifting weights with confidence. You have options when it comes to the exercises you practise and the equipment you use, and knowing these allows you to tailor your approach.

As you look to incorporate strength training into your life, it's important to remember that you don't need to know everything – nobody actually does know everything – and you can continue to learn throughout your journey. A few useful acronyms, some familiarity with common gym equipment, a selection of staple exercises and a handful of essential reminders will help you get started – and these are all covered in this chapter.

In the following pages, you will discover how to complete 22 exercises that target different muscle groups, as well as variations and form tips. These can be used to create strength training routines, refine movements you may already be familiar with, and give you the knowledge base to build your best life.

Going forwards you could try other exercises, experiment with equipment and devise your own notes to self. One truth will always stay the same: you *are* strong.

Gym Lingo

AMRAP: As many reps/rounds as possible

BB/DB/KB: Barbell/Dumbbell/Kettlebell

BMI: Body mass index

BMR: Basal metabolic rate – the energy (calories) your body requires to perform basic functions

BPM: Beats per minute

CV: Cardiovascular

DOMS: Delayed onset muscle soreness

EMOM: Every minute on the minute

HIIT: High-intensity interval training

LISS: Low-intensity steady-state exercise – cardiovascular activity at a low-to-moderate intensity

MHR: Maximum heart rate – to estimate, subtract your age from 220

PB/PR: Personal best/Personal record

ROM: Range of motion

RPE: Rate of perceived exertion – a measure of exercise intensity

TABATA: A form of interval training – 8 rounds of 20 seconds on: 10 seconds off

TUT: Time under tension

WOD: Workout of the day

You already have the strength; it's just about embracing it

Strength Training Equipment

All gym equipment is a training tool designed to target different aspects of your fitness, and you'll naturally find your preferences when it comes to what you use. Here's an overview of some of the different types:

Free Weights

Includes: Dumbbells, barbells, kettlebells, power bags, medicine balls.

Dumbbells: These can be used for most exercises, and you can even complete effective strength training sessions using just one. Dumbbell exercises often form an integral part of any long-time gym-goer's routine.

Barbells: These can hold a greater amount of weight and are more stable than dumbbells. Weight plates or "bumpers" (same-sized colourful plates) are added to the bar and collars (clips) secure them. Olympic barbells typically weigh 15 kg (33 lb) or 20 kg (44 lb) by themselves. There are also fixed-weight barbells.

Large Equipment

> **Includes:** Power cage, squat rack, lifting platform, pull-up and dip bars, benches, boxes.

Power cage: This is used in unison with a barbell for "bigger" lifts. Because you can set the hooks (the two attachments that the barbell rests on) to any height, you can perform a variety of exercises. Always set the safety bars when using a power cage.

Squat rack: This is a bit like half of a power cage and is mainly used for lower body exercises.

Machines

> **Includes:** Pin-loaded machines, plate-loaded machines, Smith machine, cables.

Pin/Plate-loaded machines: With one you use a selector pin to choose the weight, and with the other you add weight plates. Plate-loaded machines start heavier than pin-loaded ones.

Cables: These can be used to move weight through multiple planes of motion. They're very versatile and often come with a variety of different attachments.

SQUAT

Targets: Legs and core

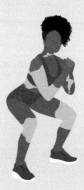

1   Stand with your feet just over hip-width apart and rotate your toes slightly outwards.

2   Keeping your core engaged and your back straight, sit backwards into your hips, bending at the knees. Ensure your feet stay planted (pressed firmly into the floor) and your head stays in line with your spine.

3   As you squat, keep your legs in line with your knees. Be careful not to let them roll inwards.

4   When you reach a comfortable depth, drive up through your feet.

SPLIT SQUAT

Targets: Legs, mainly quadriceps and glutes

1. Stand with your feet hip-width apart.
2. Take one foot backwards and sink into your back knee, allowing your front knee to bend. Ensure both knees are positioned at 90 degrees.
3. Keeping both feet where they are, drive up through your front foot.

A variation of this is a rear-foot-elevated split squat where you position your back leg on a bench or box. Depending on the placement of your front foot, you can target your quads more (closer to the bench) or your glutes (further away).

LUNGE

Targets: Legs

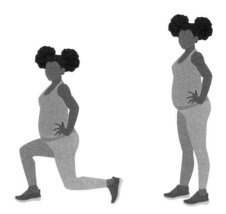

- **Rear Lunge:** Complete the same steps as a split squat (see page 131). As you drive up through your front foot, bring the leg behind you back to standing.

- **Forward Lunge:** Take your foot ahead of you rather than behind, then push off the planted foot to bring your front leg back to standing.

- **Walking Lunge:** Continue your forward lunges in a line, alternating legs.

GOOD MORNING

Targets: Legs and back, mainly hamstrings and glutes

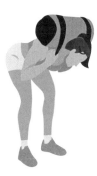

1 Stand with your feet shoulder–width apart.
2 Hinge (bend) at the hips, maintaining a soft bend in the knees and a straight back.
3 Continue pushing your hips backwards, allowing your chest to travel forwards, until you feel a stretch in your hamstrings.
4 Reverse the movement to stand back upright.

For this exercise, the weight should be positioned on your upper back.

STIFF-LEG DEADLIFT

Targets: Legs and back, mainly hamstrings and glutes

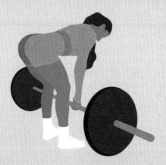

1 Stand with your feet shoulder-width apart.

2 Hinge at the hips and send your glutes backwards. Keep your core engaged and your head in line with your spine.

3 Allow your hands to trace your legs as you continue to stretch your hamstrings. Maintain a soft bend in the knees and a straight back.

4 When you reach just beyond your knees or mid-shin, drive through your feet to come back upright.

For this exercise, the weight should be in your hands close to your legs. For a single-leg variation, slowly raise one leg behind you as you hinge at the hips.

HIP THRUST

Targets: Legs, mainly glutes

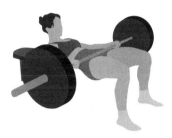

1   Sit on the floor with a bench or box.

2   Position the bench or box just below your shoulder blades, place your feet hip-width apart and rotate your toes slightly outwards.

3   Tuck your chin to your chest, engage your core and tuck your pelvis.

4   Drive through your feet to send your hips upwards. At the top position, your body should be in a straight line.

5   Squeeze your glutes and hold, then lower your hips back towards the floor.

If you're adding a weight, position this across your hips. For a single-leg variation, float one leg off the floor for the duration of the movement.

CONVENTIONAL DEADLIFT

Targets: Back, hamstrings, glutes and core

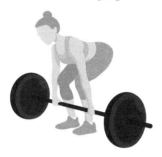

1 Stand with your feet shoulder-width apart and your lats (the "wings" of your back) tight.

2 Replicate the motion of a stiff-leg deadlift (see page 134) until your hands pass your knees.

3 At this point, bend your legs and touch the weight to the floor. If the weight knocks your knees, you likely need to hinge your hips more before bending.

4 Push the floor away with your feet as you stand up following the same path.

The best practice when picking up or dropping weights is to deadlift them.

PULL-UP

Targets: Back and biceps

- **Bodyweight Pull-Up:** Hang with your hands just over shoulder-width apart, palms facing away from you. Keep your elbows in and pull yourself towards the pull-up bar.

- **Band-Assisted Pull-Up:** Loop a resistance band around the pull-up bar and step one foot into it before pulling up. The thicker the band, the more weight it will offset, making the movement easier.

- **Eccentric/Negative Pull-Up:** Jump up to the top of the movement then slowly lower yourself back down.

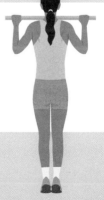

Dead hangs (hanging at the bottom of the pull-up position) and scapular shrugs (starting in a dead hang then squeezing your shoulder blades together) help develop pull-up strength.

OVERHEAD PRESS

Targets: Trapezius, triceps, front deltoids and core

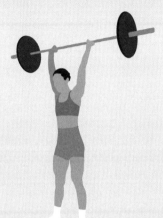

1 Stand with your feet shoulder-width apart and a slight bend in your knees.

2 Position the barbell along your upper chest with your hands just outside of your shoulders.

3 Keeping your core engaged, push the barbell up towards the ceiling until your arms are extended overhead. Move your head forwards over your spine as the barbell passes it.

4 Slowly lower the barbell back towards your chest, moving your head back to the starting position.

OVERHAND BENT-OVER ROW

Targets: Back and rear deltoids

1 Stand with your feet shoulder-width apart and the weight in your hands with your palms facing away from you.
2 Hinge at the hips, keeping your back straight, until the weight reaches your knees.
3 Engage your core, squeeze your back and keep your elbows in as you row the weight towards your belly button.
4 Slowly lower the weight back towards your knees.

For an underhand variation, replicate the movement with your palms facing towards you. Think about pulling the weight in. This also targets your biceps.

BICEP CURL

Targets: Biceps

1 Start with the weights in your hands with your palms facing towards you.
2 Relax your shoulders down and tuck your elbows into your sides.
3 Curl the weights upwards, keeping your elbows pinned to your body. Avoid swinging the weights.
4 Control the weights back down.

For a high-rep variation, practise 21s: pick a lighter weight and complete 7 reps from the bottom of the movement to the halfway point, 7 reps from the halfway point to the top, and then 7 full reps without resting in between.

HAMMER CURL

Targets: Biceps

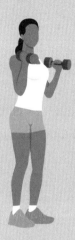

1 Stand with your feet shoulder-width apart.
2 Hold the weights in your hands at your sides with your palms facing each other.
3 Relax your shoulders down and tuck your upper arms into your torso.
4 Bend at the elbows and lift the weights towards your shoulders. Keep your wrists in line with your forearms.
5 Control the weights back down.

DUMBBELL BENCH PRESS

Targets: Chest, triceps and shoulders

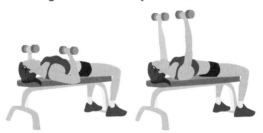

1 Holding two dumbbells to your chest, carefully lie down on a bench.

2 Press through your feet, pull your shoulder blades in and engage your core.

3 Extend your arms until the dumbbells are over your mid-chest, palms facing towards your feet.

4 Keeping your elbows in, lower the dumbbells to either side of your chest.

5 Push through your arms, chest and feet to extend your arms. Ensure the dumbbells stay in line with your chest.

Bench press or "bench" refers to the barbell variation of this exercise.

PUSH-UP

Targets: Chest, triceps, front deltoids and core

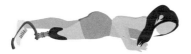

- **Bodyweight Push-Up:** Kneel on the floor, place your hands shoulder-width apart and in line with your chest, and extend your legs. Keeping your core engaged, your back straight and your head in line with your spine, lower your chest to the floor, tucking your elbows in and back. Push up through your hands.

- **Kneeling Push-Up:** Perform the same movement as above but from a kneeling position.

- **Incline Push-Up:** Instead of completing this movement from the floor, place your hands on a bench or box.

- **Eccentric/Negative Push-Up:** From kneeling or with your legs extended, slowly lower yourself to the floor, then get up however you can and reset to the starting position.

BENCH TRICEP DIP

Targets: Triceps

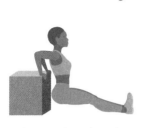 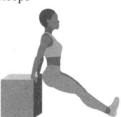

1 Sit on a bench or box.
2 Place your hands down by your hips and shift forwards until your bottom is just off the bench or box.
3 Either place your feet so your knees are at 90 degrees or extend your legs and rest on your heels.
4 Keeping your back close to and parallel with the bench, bend at your elbows and lower your hips towards the floor. Ensure your wrists stay in line with your forearms.
5 When your elbows reach 90 degrees, push up through your hands.

For a feet-elevated variation, extend your legs and rest your heels on a parallel bench. Keep your feet elevated for the duration of the movement.

STANDING
TRICEP KICKBACK

Targets: Triceps

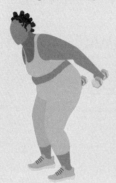

1 Stand with your feet shoulder-width apart and the weights in your hands at your sides with your palms facing each other.

2 Hinge at the hips until your hands reach your knees.

3 Keeping your elbows in, lift the weights upwards until they touch your chest.

4 Tuck your elbows into your torso and extend your forearms behind you until your shoulders, arms and wrists make a straight line.

5 Hinging at the elbows, bring the weights back towards your chest.

SHOULDER PRESS

Targets: Shoulders

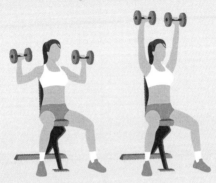

1   Adjust a bench so that you're sat one notch below upright (approximately 80 degrees) with your feet on the floor.

2   Position the weights either side of your head – you might want to "kick" them up using your knees – and angle your elbows at 90 degrees.

3   Keeping your wrists in line with your forearms, push the weights up towards the ceiling until your arms are extended overhead.

4   Lower your elbows back to 90 degrees.

The standing variation (with your feet shoulder-width apart) also targets your core.

LATERAL RAISE

Targets: Shoulders

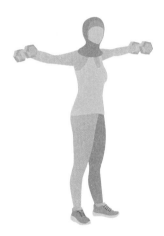

1 Stand with your feet shoulder-width apart.

2 Hold the weights in your hands at your sides with your palms facing each other.

3 Lift your arms out to your sides, slightly ahead of you with bent elbows. Pretend you're slowly flapping imaginary wings.

4 When your arms reach the point of being parallel with the floor, lower them back to your sides.

PLANK

Targets: Core, arms, back and chest

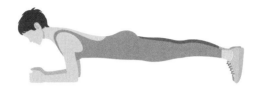

1 Kneel on the floor.

2 Rest on either your forearms set shoulder-width apart, palms flat on the floor, or on your hands. Ensure your shoulders are stacked on top of your elbows.

3 Extend your legs behind you and lower your bottom until your body creates a straight line from your head to your heels. Keep your head in line with your spine.

4 Engage your core, drawing your belly button inwards.

5 Hold this position for the desired time.

When performed correctly, most exercises will utilize your core muscles.

CRUNCHES

Targets: Core, mainly rectus abdominis
(the "six-pack" muscles)

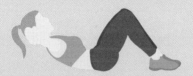

1   Lie on your back with your knees bent and your feet flat on the floor.
2   Place your hands by your sides, across your chest, or behind your ears (careful not to pull on your neck).
3   Tuck your chin to your chest and engage your core.
4   Curl your torso towards your knees, allowing your shoulder blades to lift off the floor.
5   Before the middle of your back lifts off the floor, lower your body back to the starting position.

A variation of this is a bicycle crunch: place your hands behind your ears, elevate your legs slightly and lift your shoulder blades off the floor. Then, rotating your torso, bring your opposite elbow to meet your opposite knee above your chest and continue alternating.

OBLIQUE TWIST

Targets: Core, mainly obliques

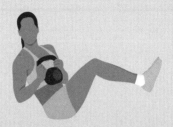

1   Sit on the floor with your knees bent and your feet together.

2   Lean backwards slightly and lift your feet off the floor, or keep them where they are.

3   Hold your hands together (or clasp a weight, such as a kettlebell or medicine ball).

4   Keep your core engaged and your shoulders back.

5   Rotate your torso to one side and lower your hands towards the floor by your hip.

6   Bring your hands back to the middle, then repeat on the other side.

LYING LEG RAISE

Targets: Core

1 Lie on the floor with your hands by your sides or tucked underneath your glutes.

2 Keeping your legs together and as straight as possible, raise them towards the ceiling.

3 When they reach 90 degrees, slowly lower them back towards the floor. Keep your core engaged and your back straight.

4 Drop your legs as far as possible without losing tension in your core.

5 At the lowest point you can reach, lift your legs back up towards the ceiling.

A variation of this is a hanging leg raise: hang from a pull-up bar and raise your legs to 90 degrees. Alternatively, you could practise hanging knee tucks: hang from a pull-up bar and tuck your knees to your chest.

Strong Reminders

Whatever stage of your strength training journey you're at, these reminders remain relevant. Keep them in mind as you pursue your fitness goals and become your strongest self.

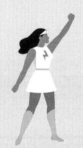

You deserve to take up space.

What you're doing counts.

Strength fluctuates – not every session will be a "good" one.

You deserve to eat (even on the days you don't exercise).

Your body needs rest.

Progress isn't always linear.

"Strong" looks different on everyone.

You're on your own journey.

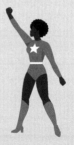

You are deserving of love, kindness and respect.

Your value is not attached to a number on the scales or your performance in the gym.

You do have the strength.

I figure if a
girl wants to
be a legend,
she should go
ahead and be one.

CALAMITY JANE

CONCLUSION

As you reach the end of this book, let's reflect on your journey so far and prepare you for your next steps.

Strength training is a tool you can use to improve your mental and physical health, heal the relationship you have with yourself and connect you with your power. It's up to you to determine how to approach your practice and what you aspire to achieve, but the key is finding what keeps you moving, motivated and committed to your goals. You deserve to feel calm in your mind, capable in your body and confident in yourself.

It's important to remember that all movement matters. You create your own definition of "strong", and there's space for every woman to succeed. Strength doesn't only lie in setting your intentions and taking action, it is also found in nurturing self-belief.

How you continue on your journey is for you to decide. You could jump straight in with a wellness regime, you could seek some additional guidance using the resources in this book, or you could read back over the pages and bookmark your favourite tips to refer to. You might want to think about your goals, start incorporating well-being practices into your routine, or hone a handful of strength training exercises to form the basis of your programme. Whatever you choose, it's essential you put your health and happiness first.

We're part of a new wave of women strengthening their minds, bodies and spirits, but we know this isn't a phase – strong is here to stay. Supported by this book, your family and friends, and other strong women, you can make this era one for the ages.

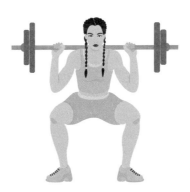

RESOURCES

Apps

Nike Training Club
StrongLifts
Strong Workout Tracker

Books

Alice Liveing, *Give Me Strength: How I Turned My Back on Restriction, Nurtured the Body I Love, and How You Can Too* (2024)

Dr Hazel Wallace, *The Female Factor: Making Women's Health Count – and What it Means for You* (2022)

Poorna Bell, *Stronger: Changing Everything I Knew About Women's Strength* (2021)

Tally Rye, *Train Happy: An Intuitive Exercise Plan for Every Body* (2020)

Charities

Her Sport – www.hersport.ie
This Girl Can – www.thisgirlcan.co.uk
Women in Sport – www.womeninsport.org
Women's Sports Foundation – www.womenssportsfoundation.org

Websites

Girls Gone Strong – www.girlsgonestrong.com
PureGym Exercise Guides – www.puregym.com
Squat University – www.squatuniversity.com
Strength Level – www.strengthlevel.com
Women's Health – www.womenshealthmag.com

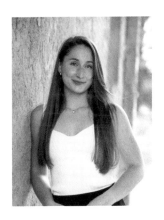

About the Author

Saffron Hooton is an author, editor and fitness influencer from West Sussex. She has been strength training for six years, practises pole fitness and dance, and is a qualified Exercise to Music Instructor. As a Women's Best Athlete, Saffron creates health and fitness content for her Instagram account, @saff_fit. *Strong Woman Era* brings together Saffron's passions for strength training, writing and female empowerment.

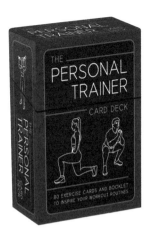

The Personal Trainer Card Deck

ISBN: 978-1-83799-493-9

GET STRONGER, FEEL FITTER
AND BE MORE ACTIVE

Complete with 70 exercise cards and 10 workout challenges, this deck and booklet will help make fitness fun! Create unique, effective and invigorating training routines to develop strength and improve your cardiovascular fitness. Simply shuffle the deck, select five cards and get started!

Image Credits

Have you enjoyed this book?
If so, why not write a review on
your favourite website?

If you're interested in finding out more about
our books, find us on Facebook at Summersdale
Publishers, on Twitter/X at @Summersdale and
on Instagram and TikTok at @summersdalebooks
and get in touch. We'd love to hear from you!

Thanks very much for buying
this Summersdale book.

www.summersdale.com

"This is an amazing guide for women who are new to or are less confident with strength training. Strong Woman Era will help boost your self-belief and aids in the breakdown of myths and stereotypes that women face."

Olivia Broome, double Paralympic medallist, parapowerlifting @oliviabroomepowerlifter

"Strong Woman Era is a lovely little book, full of positive affirmations, sound fitness advice and, most importantly, it offers a reassuring voice that any woman can be a strong woman. I loved it!"

Rachel Lawrence, Pilates instructor and author @thegirlwiththepilatesmat

"This is the book I needed to read at the start of my strength training journey 30 years ago! Straightforward, easy to digest and beautifully illustrated throughout, Strong Woman Era is a powerhouse of information."

Jacqueline Hooton, personal trainer, active-ageing advocate and author @hergardengym

"It is brilliant to see women's strength training entering the mainstream, with more and more women claiming back their right to sport and exercise. Strong Woman Era by Saffron Hooton empowers all women to build healthy foundations for their later lives."

Women in Sport, UK charity